Copyright © 2021

Contents

What is peptic ulcer disease? 8

Who is more likely to get ulcers? 8

SYMPTOMS AND CAUSES......................9

What causes ulcers?......................9

H. pylori bacteria 9

Pain relievers 11

Rare causes 13

Can coffee and spicy foods cause ulcers? 14

What are some ulcer symptoms? 14

DIAGNOSIS AND TESTS 16

How are ulcers diagnosed?......................16

Endoscopy 16

H. Pylori tests......................17

Imaging tests 17

MANAGEMENT AND TREATMENT......................18

Will ulcers heal on their own?.....................18

What ulcer treatments are available? 18

PREVENTION......................................20

How can I prevent ulcers? 20

OUTLOOK / PROGNOSIS.........................21

Are ulcers curable? 21

How long does it take an ulcer to heal? 21

LIVING WITH 22

Will drinking milk help an ulcer? 22

Is it safe to take antacids? 22

What should ulcer patients eat?.................23

What questions should I ask my doctor?......23

Ulcer Diet 24

Benefits..25

How It Works 28

Duration 29

What to Eat 30

Compliant Foods 30

Non-Compliant Foods 31

Best Choices 32

Foods to Limit 35

Recommended Timing 37

Cooking Tips 37

Modifications 38

Considerations 39

General Nutrition 39

Practicality 39

Energy and Health 40

ULCER DIET RECIPES 40

SJ Trail Munch 40

Gingered Butternut Squash Soup 42

Broccoli Soup 45

Potato Soup 47

CABBAGE-CARROT-APPLE JUICE 50

GOLDEN DARK CHOCOLATE TRUFFLES 51

Healthy Chicken and Mushroom Stew 54

Banana and Nutella heaven 58

Sunda Vathal Podi | Sundakkai Vathal Podi 60

TAPIOCA PUDDING 63

Cabbage Carrot Juice 65

Egg Salad Makeover 67

Kale Salad 69

Chicken Noodle Soup (Bland Diet) 72

CREAMY POTATO SOUP 74

CARROT GINGER SOUP 76

Green Cabbage Juice 79

Alkalizing Celery Lemonade 81

Cabbage juice 82

Cranberry Coulis Recipe 84

Carrot and Kale Quinoa Patties [Vegan]........86

Raw Purple Sauerkraut [Vegan] 90

Cinnamon Spiced Apple and Grape Salad [Vegan]........................98

Instant Pot Cabbage Soup 101

Matcha Berry Pancakes 103

Hazelnut Mousse With Warm Raspberries 107

Baked Kale Chips........................110

Homemade Kimchi........................112

Waldorf salad 117

Sautéed Mackerel 119

Celery Juice 121

Cabbage Carrot Apple Juice 123

Cabbage Cucumber Melon Juice 124

Cabbage Beetroot Orange Juice.................. 125

High-fibre muesli..................................... 126

Soft herb scrambled egg with asparagus 128

What is peptic ulcer disease?

Peptic ulcer disease is a condition in which painful sores or ulcers develop in the lining of the stomach or the first part of the small intestine (the duodenum). Normally, a thick layer of mucus protects the stomach lining from the effect of its digestive juices. But many things can reduce this protective layer, allowing stomach acid to damage the tissue.

Who is more likely to get ulcers?

One in 10 people develops an ulcer. Risk factors that make ulcers more likely include:

• Frequent use of nonsteroidal anti-inflammatory drugs (NSAIDs), a group of common pain relievers that includes ibuprofen (Advil® or Motrin®).

- A family history of ulcers.

- Illness such as liver, kidney or lung disease.

- Regularly drinking alcohol.

- Smoking.

SYMPTOMS AND CAUSES

What causes ulcers?

People used to think that stress or certain foods could cause ulcers. But researchers haven't found any evidence to support those theories. Instead, studies have revealed two main causes of ulcers:

- Helicobacter pylori (H. pylori) bacteria.

- Pain-relieving NSAID medications.

H. pylori bacteria

H. pylori commonly infects the stomach. About 50% of the world's population has an H. pylori infection, often without any symptoms. Researchers believe people can transmit H. pylori from person to person, especially during childhood.

The H. pylori bacteria stick to the layer of mucus in the digestive tract and cause inflammation (irritation), which can cause this protective lining to break down. This breakdown is a problem because your stomach contains strong acid intended to digest food. Without the mucus layer to protect it, the acid can eat into stomach tissue.

However, for most people the presence of H. pylori doesn't have a negative impact. Only 10%

to 15% of people with H. pylori end up developing ulcers .

Pain relievers

Another major cause of peptic ulcer disease is the use of NSAIDs, a group of medications used to relieve pain. NSAIDS can wear away at the mucus layer in the digestive tract. These medications have the potential to cause peptic ulcers to form:

• Aspirin (even those with a special coating).

• Naproxen (Aleve®, Anaprox®, Naprosyn® and others).

• Ibuprofen (Motrin®, Advil®, Midol® and others).

- Prescription NSAIDs (Celebrex®, Cambia® and others).

Acetaminophen (Tylenol®) is not an NSAID and won't cause damage to your stomach. People who can't take NSAIDs are often directed to take acetaminophen.

Not everyone who takes NSAIDs will develop ulcers. NSAID use coupled with an H. pylori infection is potentially the most dangerous. People who have H. pylori and who frequently use NSAIDs are more likely to have damage to the mucus layer, and their damage can be more severe. Developing an ulcer from NSAID use also increases if you:

- Take high doses of NSAIDs.

- Are 70 years or older.

- Are female.

- Use corticosteroids (drugs your doctor might prescribe for asthma, arthritis or lupus) at the same time as taking NSAIDs.

- Use NSAIDS continuously for a long time.

- Have a history of ulcer disease.

Rare causes

Infrequently, other situations cause peptic ulcer disease. People may develop ulcers after:

- Being seriously ill from various infections or diseases.

- Having surgery.

- Taking other medications, such as steroids.

Peptic ulcer disease can also occur if you have a rare condition called Zollinger-Ellison syndrome (gastrinoma). This condition forms a tumor of acid-producing cells in the digestive tract. These tumors can be cancerous or noncancerous. The cells produce excessive amounts of acid that damages stomach tissue.

Can coffee and spicy foods cause ulcers?

It's a common misconception that coffee and spicy foods can cause ulcers. In the past, you might have heard that people with ulcers should eat a bland diet. But now we know that if you have an ulcer, you can still enjoy whatever foods you choose as long as they don't make your symptoms worse.

What are some ulcer symptoms?

Some people with ulcers don't experience any symptoms. But signs of an ulcer can include:

- Gnawing or burning pain in your middle or upper stomach between meals or at night.

- Pain that temporarily disappears if you eat something or take an antacid.

- Bloating.

- Heartburn.

- Nausea or vomiting.

In severe cases, symptoms can include:

- Dark or black stool (due to bleeding).

- Vomiting.

- Weight loss.

- Severe pain in your mid- to upper abdomen.

DIAGNOSIS AND TESTS

How are ulcers diagnosed?

Your healthcare provider may be able to make the diagnosis just by talking with you about your symptoms. If you develop an ulcer and you're not taking NSAIDs, the cause is likely an H. pylori infection. To confirm the diagnosis, you'll need one of these tests:

Endoscopy

If you have severe symptoms, your provider may recommend an upper endoscopy to determine if you have an ulcer. In this procedure, the doctor inserts an endoscope (a small, lighted tube with a tiny camera) through your throat and into your stomach to look for abnormalities.

H. Pylori tests

Tests for H. pylori are now widely used and your provider will tailor treatment to reduce your symptoms and kill the bacteria. A breath test is the easiest way to discover H. pylori. Your provider can also look for it with a blood or stool test, or by taking a sample during an upper endoscopy.

Imaging tests

Less frequently, imaging tests such as X-rays and CT scans are used to detect ulcers. You have to drink a specific liquid that coats the digestive tract and makes ulcers more visible to the imaging machines.

MANAGEMENT AND TREATMENT

Will ulcers heal on their own?

Though ulcers can sometimes heal on their own, you shouldn't ignore the warning signs. Without the right treatment, ulcers can lead to serious health problems, including:

• Bleeding.

• Perforation (a hole through the wall of the stomach).

• Gastric outlet obstruction (from swelling or scarring) that blocks the passageway from the stomach to the small intestine.

What ulcer treatments are available?

If your ulcer is bleeding, your doctor may treat it during an endoscopy procedure by injecting medications into it. Your doctor could also use a clamp or cauterization (burning tissue) to seal it off and stop the bleeding.

For most people, doctors treat ulcers with medications, including:

• Proton pump inhibitors (PPI): These drugs reduce acid, which allows the ulcer to heal. PPIs include Prilosec®, Prevacid®, Aciphex®, Protonix® and Nexium®.

• Histamine receptor blockers (H2 blockers): These drugs also reduce acid production and include Tagamet®, Pepcid®, Zantac® and Axid®.

• Antibiotics: These medications kill bacteria. Doctors use them to treat H. pylori.

• Protective medications: Like a liquid bandage, these medications cover the ulcer in a protective layer to prevent further damage from digestive acids and enzymes. Doctors commonly recommend Carafate® or Pepto-Bismol®.

PREVENTION

How can I prevent ulcers?

You may be able to prevent ulcers from forming if you:

• Talk to your doctor about alternatives to NSAID medications (like acetaminophen) to relieve pain.

• Discuss protective measures with your doctor, if you can't stop taking an NSAID.

- Opt for the lowest effective dose of NSAID and take it with a meal.

- Quit smoking.

- Drink alcohol in moderation, if at all.

OUTLOOK / PROGNOSIS

Are ulcers curable?

For most people, treatment that targets the underlying cause (usually H. pylori bacterial infection or NSAID use) is effective at eliminating peptic ulcer disease. Ulcers can reoccur, though, especially if H. pylori isn't fully cleared from your system or you continue to smoke or use NSAIDs.

How long does it take an ulcer to heal?

It generally takes several weeks of treatment for an ulcer to heal.

LIVING WITH

Will drinking milk help an ulcer?

No. Milk may temporarily soothe ulcer pain because it coats the stomach lining. But milk also causes your stomach to produce more acid and digestive juices, which can make ulcers worse.

Is it safe to take antacids?

Antacids temporarily relieve ulcer symptoms. However, they can interfere with the effectiveness of prescribed medications. Check with your doctor to find out if antacids are safe to take while undergoing treatment.

What should ulcer patients eat?

No foods have been proven to negatively or positively impact ulcers. However, eating a nutritious diet and getting enough exercise and sleep is good for your overall health.

What questions should I ask my doctor?

If you have stomach ulcers, you may want to ask your doctor:

- What pain reliever can I use instead of an NSAID?

- How will I know if the H. pylori infection is gone?

- How do we find out if the ulcer has healed?

- What can I do relieve symptoms at home during treatment?

Ulcer Diet

An ulcer diet is intended to help reduce the pain and irritation that comes from a peptic ulcer—a painful sore that develops on the lining of your stomach, esophagus, or small intestine. Your doctor may put you on medication for your condition, but following an ulcer diet is an essential part of your overall care plan to manage symptoms and help your ulcer heal.

Foods or beverages don't cause ulcers, nor can they cure them. However, certain foods (e.g., fermented dairy foods) can help repair damaged tissue, and those that perpetuate acid build-up and inflammation (e.g., fried choices) may further aggravate your ulcer and threaten your digestive tract's natural layer of protection.

An ulcer diet is appropriate for anyone with an ulcer. It can also help those with gastritis or general stomach irritation.

Benefits

Your doctor is far more likely to treat your ulcer with medications instead of diet alone, but adding an ulcer diet to your treatment can definitely help you feel better faster and possibly prevent another ulcer in the future.

Following an ulcer diet along with other treatment recommendations your doctor suggests can be beneficial because it can:

• Correct any nutritional deficiencies that may be contributing to your symptoms

- Provide the protein and other nutrients your body needs to heal

- Help you eliminate foods that aggravate the lining of your stomach or small intestine

- Help to control related conditions like Crohn's disease, celiac disease, or bacterial infections, which might be contributing to your ulcer

Most peptic ulcers are caused by long-term use of nonsteroidal anti-inflammatory drugs (NSAIDs), which can erode gastrointestinal lining, or by a bacterial infection known as Helicobacter pylori (H. pylori). An ulcer diet addresses both of these by including certain foods that have antibacterial properties and compounds that help promote healing.

A 2015 review published in The World Journal of Gastroenterology looked at the use of polyphenols, a type of antioxidant compound in many plant foods, to manage peptic ulcers. The authors identified a wide range of polyphenols from foods like apples, grapes, green tea, pomegranates, turmeric, berries, and peanuts that can be beneficial in ulcer management.

Some of the polyphenols helped to heal the stomach erosions faster, and others had antibacterial effects and helped kill H. pylori. The polyphenols in green tea suppressed some of the compounds that trigger inflammation and helped to strengthen the mucosal lining of the stomach.

While spices that add heat to foods are not typically advised on an ulcer diet, a review of studies on diet and H. pylori found that some spices that simply add flavor also help kill the bacteria. Other foods that showed an antibacterial effect include fermented dairy foods like kefir or yogurt.

There's also evidence that honey, especially manuka honey, can kill H. pylori and other bacteria. Of course, there are other possible causes of peptic ulcers as well, and an ulcer diet targets two additional ones in particular—poor nutrition and excessive alcohol use.

How It Works

An ulcer diet works by helping to promote healing, avoiding irritation to the lining of your stomach or duodenum, and limiting excess acid production.

There are no strict rules about which foods to eat, but try to add as many foods as you can from the best choices list, and definitely avoid foods that make you feel worse or trigger excess acid production and reflux.

Eating enough protein is also important. While your ulcer is healing, aim for about 1.2 grams of protein per kilogram of your ideal body weight. The remainder of your calories should come from high fiber carbs like legumes, whole grains, fruits, and vegetables.

A higher-fiber diet is associated with a lower risk of peptic ulcers. The report also advises adding some zinc and selenium to help with healing.

Duration

You should stay on an ulcer diet until your doctor tells you your ulcer is completely healed. Afterward, you can resume your normal way of eating. However, if you feel better while on the diet or you have risk factors for ulcers, like smoking, this way of eating may be worth continuing—even if in a modified way.

What to Eat

Compliant Foods

- Fruits (any, fresh or frozen)

- Vegetables

- Legumes

- Lean meats (e.g.,skinless poultry, lean beef)

- Fish and seafood

- Eggs

- Whole soy foods (e.g., tofu or tempeh)

- Fermented dairy foods (e.g., kefir or yogurt)

- Healthy fats like olive oil, avocados, and nuts

- Whole and cracked grains

- Green tea

- Herbs and spices (mild; fresh or dried)

Non-Compliant Foods

- Alcohol

- Coffee (regular, decaf)

- Caffeinated foods and drinks

- Milk or cream

- Fatty meats

- Fried foods/high-fat foods

- Heavily spiced foods

- Salty foods

- Citrus fruits and juices

- Tomatoes/tomato products

- Chocolate

Best Choices

Fruits: Any fresh or frozen fruits are good and contribute beneficial fiber and antioxidants. Berries, apples, grapes, and pomegranates are among the best choices for ulcer healing polyphenols. If citrus fruits or juices like orange or grapefruit trigger reflux, avoid those.

Vegetables: Leafy greens, bright red and orange vegetables, and cruciferous vegetables like broccoli, cauliflower, and kale are packed with vitamins and antioxidants that are especially good for your overall health and healing. Avoid spicy peppers and tomatoes/tomato products if they cause reflux. Limit raw vegetables, as they can be harder to digest.

Lean proteins: Skinless poultry, lean beef like sirloin or tenderloin, fish, eggs, tofu, tempeh, dry beans, and peas are excellent sources of low-fat protein. Fatty fish like salmon, mackerel, and sardines provide omega-3 fats, which can reduce inflammation and may be helpful in preventing another ulcer.

Fermented dairy: Products like kefir and Greek yogurt provide probiotics along with protein, so they're good choices.

Breads and grains: 100% whole grain breads and whole or cracked grains like oats, quinoa, farro, millet, or sorghum are good sources of fiber to include in your diet.

Herbs and spices: You can use most mild herbs and spices liberally. They're all concentrated sources of health-promoting antioxidants. Best bets include turmeric, cinnamon, ginger, and garlic, which have antimicrobial and anti-inflammatory properties. For a sweetener, try to use honey instead of sugar.

Foods to Limit

Alcohol: All alcohol is a stomach irritant and will delay healing. Avoid wine, beer, and spirits.

Caffeine: You should cut back or eliminate coffee, tea, and caffeinated sodas, as these can increase stomach acid production.

Milk: Milk used to be recommended as a treatment for ulcers, but the latest research has found that it increases stomach acid, so it's best to avoid it.

Certain meats: Avoid highly-seasoned meats, lunch meats, sausages, and any fried or fatty meats and proteins.

High-fat foods: Try to avoid large amounts of added fats, which can increase stomach acid and trigger reflux. You may need to avoid gravy, cream soups, and highly-seasoned salad dressings. (Healthy fats are OK.)

Spicy foods: You may want to skip anything that is "hot" such as chili peppers, horseradish, black pepper, and sauces and condiments that contain them, especially if they bother you or cause any pain or reflux.

Salty foods: Researchers have found that highly salted foods may promote the growth of H. pylori. Be aware that pickles, olives, and other brined or fermented vegetables are high in salt and are associated with an increased risk of H. pylori ulcers.

Chocolate: Chocolate can increase stomach acid production, and some people find that it triggers reflux symptoms.

Recommended Timing

Try to eat five or six small meals each day, rather than three large ones. Stomach acid is produced every time you eat, but large meals require much more of it for digestion, which can be irritating.

Finish up eating at least three hours before bedtime, and try to stay upright for a few hours after your last bite for improved digestion and less acid reflux.

Cooking Tips

Stick to lower fat cooking methods like roasting, braising, and grilling instead of frying. Also, limit your use of butter and oils when you cook, as these can be harder to digest.

Modifications

In some cases, celiac disease or inflammatory bowel diseases can be associated with ulcers. If you have another health condition that affects your stomach or intestinal tract, it's important that you adhere to those diet recommendations as well as an ulcer diet.

For celiac disease, that means eating only gluten-free grains like quinoa, millet, sorghum, or rice, and taking care to read food labels for sources of hidden gluten.

For inflammatory bowel diseases, this might mean limiting lactose-containing foods, choosing lower-fiber foods, and avoiding things like carbonated beverages.

Considerations

When adopting the ulcer management diet, these factors may come into play.

General Nutrition

An ulcer diet should not have a negative impact on your nutrition status. As long as you maintain good variety in your diet, any nutrients the foods you are limiting contain will be provided by other foods.

If you're trying to add more polyphenol-rich foods and fiber to your diet, and cutting back on fatty foods, an ulcer diet may be even more nutritious than your regular diet.

Practicality

It should be fairly easy to stick with an ulcer diet when you're preparing your own meals at home.

However, it might be challenging to stay on track when you're traveling, attending parties, or celebrating holidays. If you can't pass up that glass of wine or piece of chocolate cake, make it a small one.

Energy and Health

With fast food, chips, and alcohol off-limits, you might find that you're eating healthier, feeling better, and maybe even dropping some weight.

ULCER DIET RECIPES

In this part are ulcer diet recipes to help keep your ulcer at bay

SJ Trail Munch

Preparation time

5 minutes

Ingredients

- 1 cup dry roasted peanuts

- 1 cup raw almonds

- 1 cup shelled pecan halves

- 1 cup Peanut M & M candies

- 1 cup shelled, raw pistachios

- 3/4 cup sunflower seeds

Instructions

1. Mix all ingredients together and store in an air-tight container on the counter.

2. One handful is about two tablespoons

Gingered Butternut Squash Soup

Preparation time

50 minutes

INGREDIENTS

- 1 tablespoon coconut oil

- 1 onion* (optional)

- 1 tablespoon ginger (chopped)

- 5 cups butternut squash (chopped)

- 2.5 cups coconut milk (from the can, not the watery stuff in the box)

- 2.5 cups water

- 1 ripe apple (about 1 cup)

- 2 tablespoons Daily Turmeric Tonic

- 3 heaping tablespoons (3 scoops) Further Food Collagen

INSTRUCTIONS

1. Heat coconut oil in soup pot. Add diced onion and a pinch of salt and saute until translucent (about 5 minutes).

2. Add ginger and Daily Turmeric Tonic and cook for 2 minutes.

3. Add chopped butternut squash.*

4. Add coconut milk and water, bring to a boil and then reduce heat to a simmer.

5. Add the apples after about 10 minutes.

6. Cook an additional 5 minutes, until squash and fruit are soft.

7. Add Collagen, blend, and taste for salt.

Broccoli Soup

Preparation time

35 minutes

Ingredients

- 2 tbsp coconut oil

- 1 small onion, chopped

- 2 cloves garlic, minced

- 1 tsp ground cumin (or more, to taste)

- 1 large head broccoli, cut in chunks (including stalk)

- 2 cups chopped Swish chard or spinach

- 4 cups homemade bone broth or stock

- ¼ cup probiotic yogurt plus extra for decoration

• salt and black pepper to taste

Instructions

1. In a large pot heat the coconut oil over medium heat.

2. Add the onion and cook for 4-5 minutes or until softened and translucent.

3. Add the garlic and cook for 30 seconds.

4. Add the broccoli, cumin and bone broth and bring the soup to a low boil.

5. Cover with a lid and cook for 10-15 minutes or until the broccoli is fork tender.

6. Add the Swish chard and cook until just wilted.

7. Using an immersion blender or food processor or blender, puree the soup until smooth.

8. Stir in the yogurt.

9. Season to taste with salt and black pepper.

10. Serve warm.

Potato Soup

Preparation time

20 minutes

Ingredients

- 2 small sweet potatoes

- 1 cup vegetable broth

- 1 carrot

- 1 avocado

- 1 cup spinach

- Salt to taste

Instructions

1. Wash and peel potatoes.

2. Chop into cubes and press.

3. Wash, cut and press carrot.

4. Slice avocado in half.

5. Remove the pit and scoop the flesh out.

6. Mix with broth and press.

7. Transfer about ½ of the pulp into pot.

8. Add squeezed juice and a pinch of salt.

9. On medium heat bring to a boil.

10. Stir until everything is nicely combined.

11. Wash and press spinach.

12. Combine spinach juice and pulp, stir until smooth, and warm it lightly.

13. Pour into the middle of each soup and serve.

CABBAGE-CARROT-APPLE JUICE

Preparation time

15 minutes

INGREDIENTS

- ¼ head of cabbage, tough stem cut out

- 1 large carrot, peeled

- 1 small organic apple, any variety

- Add ¼ tsp cinnamon for added heart health

INSTRUCTIONS

1. Using a commercial juicer, place an 8-ounce glass beneath the spout and insert vegetables one-by-one until all juice has dispensed from juicer.

2. Mix and drink immediately.

GOLDEN DARK CHOCOLATE TRUFFLES

Preparation time

1 hour 30 minutes

Ingredients:

- 3/4 cup cashew butter

- 1/4 cup almond flour

- 2 tsp. blackstrap molasses (or substitute maple syrup)

- 1 teaspoon maple syrup (optional but makes the truffles sweeter)

- 2 teaspoons coconut oil, melted

- 1/2 teaspoon turmeric powder*

- 1/4 teaspoon ginger powder*

- pinch of black pepper*

- OR 3/4 teaspoon Golden Milk Spice Blend from Spice Sanctuary*

- 1/2 teaspoon ground cardamom

- 40 grams good-quality organic dark chocolate, melted

Instructions

1. To make the truffle filling, mix cashew butter, almond flour, and molasses in a bowl using a fork or electric whisk.

2. In another bowl, combine the coconut oil and spices and mix well before adding into the cashew butter mixture and folding it in thoroughly.

3. Take a small spoonful into your hand and roll the mixture into a round ball, approximately half an inch in diameter, and place on baking parchment on a tray.

4. Repeat until all the mixture has been rolled.

5. Chill in the fridge for 30 minutes.

6. Melt the chocolate in a bowl.

7. Using a spoon, dip the truffles into the melted chocolate before returning to the tray again.

8. Repeat until all the truffles have been covered in chocolate.

9. Refrigerate for another 30 minutes and serve.

Healthy Chicken and Mushroom Stew

Preparation time

45 minutes

INGREDIENTS

• 5 chicken pieces

- 4 large mushrooms (chopped)

- 1 red bell pepper

- 1 cup spinach (chopped)

- 1 onion

- 2 cloves garlic

- 1 maggi cube

- 1 chicken stock cube

- 1 tsp mild curry powder

- 1 tsp dried thyme

- 1/4 tsp salt (taste before adding salt)

- 1 tbsp olive oil

INSTRUCTIONS

1. Blend the bell pepper with a little water to help the blender blend and then set aside.

2. Prepare all the ingredients: chop the onion, garlic mushrooms, spinach and set aside.

3. Wash your chicken and set aside.

4. Heat the oil in a large pan over medium heat and add the chopped onion and garlic.

5. Saute for 30 seconds and then add the chopped mushrooms and cook until mushrooms are soft

6. Add the seasoning: crush maggi cube and chicken stock cube over the frying vegetables, add curry powder, dried thyme and salt.

7. Mix everything together and keep frying!

8. The mushrooms should keep the mixture wet however turn down the heat if it gets a little dry and cover with a lid

9. After about 2 minutes, add the blended pepper, stir, replace the lid and simmer on low heat for 10 minutes or until the water reduce.

10. After 10 minutes, the water should have reduced and everything should look more like a paste, add the chicken pieces and really mix everything together ensuring that the sauce completely coats each chicken piece.

11. Mix in a 1/4 cup water and cover the pot, simmer on low heat for 10 minutes.

12. After 10 minutes mix in 3/4 cups water, cover the pot and simmer on low heat for a

further 30 minutes or until chicken juices run clear

13. After 30 minutes, add the chopped spinach and cook for a further 2 minutes.

14. Mix once more and serve with rice or baked potatoes or boiled yam

Banana and Nutella heaven

Preparation time

15 minutes

Ingredients

1 teaspoon nutella

1 banana

2 wheat bread slices

Instructions

1. Toast wheat bread until light brown (I prefer mines a little burnt).

2. Let it cool for 2 minutes or if you have no patience like me, put the bread in the freezer for about a minute.

3. Cut banana into slices.

4. Remove bread from freezer, and spread nutella on the bread with a butter knife or spatula.

5. Add banana slices on top on nutella covered bread and add top slice.

6. Enjoy!

Sunda Vathal Podi | Sundakkai Vathal Podi

Preparation time

15 minutes

Ingredients

To dry roast

- 2 Tblsp chana dhal or kadala paruppu

- 1 Tblsp urid dhal

- 1 Tblsp coriander seeds

- 1/2 tsp cumin seeds

- 1/4 tsp asafoetida

- handful of curry leaves

- To fry in oil

- 1/2 tsp pepper

- 1/4 cup sundakkai vathal

Instructions

1. Heat a pan.

2. Add chana dhal, urid dhal, coriander seeds, cumin and curry leaves.

3. Roast in medium or low flame till it becomes golden brown.

4. Add asafoetida and transfer the things to a plate.

5. Let everything get cooled down.

6. Heat oil in a pan.

7. Add pepper and sundakkai vathal.

8. Fry it till it becomes crispy.

9. Transfer it to a plate and cool it.

10. Take the dry roasted ingredients in a blender and powder them finely.

11. Add fried sundakka and pepper to them and grind once again.

12. Cool the powder and transfer it to a bottle or ziplock cover.

13. Tasty sundakka vathal podi will be ready in very few minutes.

TAPIOCA PUDDING

Preparation time

1 hour 20 minutes

INGREDIENTS

- ¼ cup tapioca pearls

- ½ coconut milk

- 1 tablespoon coconut sugar or maple syrup

- 1 teaspoon cinnamon

- 1 teaspoon ginger, grated

- 1 teaspoon Himalayan sea salt

- 1 mango, sliced

- 1 scoop Sunwarrior Classic Plus protein (to be added while serving)

Instructions

1. Using a small pan, heat up the coconut milk and tapioca pearls for about 10–15 minutes.

2. Slowly add cinnamon, sugar, ginger, and sea salt to the mixture.

3. Keep stirring until all ingredients are mixed well.

4. Transfer the ingredients to a glass bowl, and store in the refrigerator for an hour before serving.

5. Slice the mango into small squares, and serve it a topping for the dish.

Cabbage Carrot Juice

Preparation time

15 minutes

Ingredients:

1/2 cabbage

1 lemon

2 medium-sized beets

4 medium-sized carrots

Instructions:

1. Wash carrot and cut into appropriate sizes.

2. The beet should be washed, and then peeled before cutting.

3. Wash lemon with baking soda, and prepare by cutting with the peel intact.

4. Wash cabbage thoroughly and cut into appropriate sizes.

5. Put lever on "close." Alternate the order of ingredient insertion.

Egg Salad Makeover

Preparation time

10 minutes

Ingredients

- Hard Boiled Eggs

- Mayo alternative such as Nayonaise

- tsp of Curry powder

- pinch of cayenne pepper (just a pinch, really!)

- Lemon juice to taste (about 1 tbsp)

- Cucumber

- Broccoli Sprouts

- Pita of choice

Instructions

1. Chop or slice eggs in an egg slicer and place in a mixing bowl

2. Add desired amount of Mayo, Curry, Cayenne, and lemon.

3. Spread out on a Pita with cucumber slices and sprouts.

Kale Salad

Preparation time

30 minutes

INGREDIENTS

- 1 large bunch of kale (either curly or Tuscan is fine. I like both)

- 1/3 cup pumpkin seeds

- 1/2 cup broccoli sprouts

- 1/4 cup lemon juice

- 1/3 cup tahini

- 1 clove garlic

- 3 Tbsp* olive oil (60ml)

- 1 – 2 Tbsp water (20ml – 40ml)

- 1/4 tsp salt + extra for the kale

Instructions

1. To prepare the kale – wash and cut the leaves off each hard stem

2. Gather the leaves together and cut into thin strips (like coleslaw)

3. Sprinkle with a little salt (about 1/2 tsp) and massage until the kale becomes soft. This will be about 3 or so minutes

4. Set the kale aside and prepare the dressing

5. Place the lemon juice, tahini, garlic, olive oil and 1/4 tsp salt in the Thermomix (or a food processor).

6. Blend until the dressing is creamy (15 secs, speed 6).

7. Scrape down the sides of the bowl, then blend again, 10 secs speed 2 and slowly drizzle in the water until it's a nice, slightly runny, dressing. You may not need all of it.

8. You can also just stir all these ingredients together in a bowl if you'd prefer.

9. Just make sure it's a little runny, as a dressing should be, and you mince the garlic beforehand

10. Pour the dressing over the salad, add in the pumpkin seeds and broccoli sprouts then toss to combine

11. This goes perfectly with grilled or baked meats, but is also delicious when served with a poached egg or two.

12. Enjoy!

Chicken Noodle Soup (Bland Diet)

Preparation time

20 minutes

INGREDIENTS

• 2 Knorr Chicken Stock Cups

- 10 Cups water

- 6 oz. No Yolk Egg Noodles

- 1 Can sliced carrots, drained & rinsed

- 1 10.75 oz. chicken in water, drained

- Thyme

Instructions

1. Boil water, add chicken stock cups.

2. When dissolved, add Egg Noodles.

3. When tender, add canned chicken & carrots and Thyme.

4. Simmer until heated through and flavor has distributed through the soup.

CREAMY POTATO SOUP

Preparation time

40 minutes

INGREDIENTS

- 6 medium potatoes, peeled and chopped

- 5 cups filtered water

- 1 bay leaf

- 1 sage leaf

- 1/8 teaspoon dried or 1/2 teaspoon fresh thyme

- 1 sprig fresh cilantro

- 1 tablespoon organic, non-GMO miso paste

- 2 cups non-dairy milk

- Freshly-ground black pepper

INSTRUCTIONS

1. Place the potatoes and water in a large pot.

2. Add the bay leaf, sage, thyme, miso, and cilantro and bring to a boil.

3. Reduce heat to medium-low.

4. Cover and simmer until the potatoes have softened, about 30 minutes.

5. Remove the potatoes from the pot and puree in a food processor until smooth or, place

potatoes in a bowl and mash with a potato masher or a hand blender until smooth.

6. Return the potatoes to pot.

7. Stir in the non-dairy milk and ground pepper. Simmer for another 8 minutes and serve.

CARROT GINGER SOUP

Preparation time

35 minutes

INGREDIENTS

- 500 g carrots, peeled and chopped

- 1 medium potato, peeled and chopped

- 1 medium yellow onion, chopped

- 4 garlic cloves, diced

- 1 cm piece ginger root, peeled and chopped

- 6 cups (1.5L) water

- 1/4 cup smooth or crunchy natural peanut butter

- 1/4 tsp sea salt

INSTRUCTIONS

1. Saute the garlic, fresh ginger and onion in a big pot with 2 Tbsp of olive oil for 5'.

2. Then add the carrots, the potatoes and cover with water.

3. Bring to the boil then reduce the heat to medium-low.

4. Cook for 20-30' until the carrots are tender.

5. Allow to cool before transferring to a food processor.

6. Remove ½ cup of cooking liquid so you can adjust the consistency to your taste.

7. Add the peanut butter and blend until smooth.

8. Serve with spicy chickpeas.

Green Cabbage Juice

Preparation time

15 minutes

Ingredients

- green cabbage 1.22 oz (2 Medium leaves)

- green apple 8 oz (1 1/3 medium apples)

- chard 2.33 oz (1 1/2 leaves)

- kale 1.9 oz (3/4 cup, chopped)

- celery 1.33 oz (1 medium stalk)

- lemon 1.78 oz (1 small lemon)

Instructions

1. Wash all produce.

2. Make sure all of the dirt is removed from the kale and chard before putting it in your juicer.

3. Cut the lemon and place directly in the press.

4. If you do not have a juice press, peel and juice with the rest of the ingredients.

5. Grind and press the remaining ingredients together.

Alkalizing Celery Lemonade

Preparation time

15 minutes

Ingredients

- 1 bunch celery 10-12 oz.

- 2 Tbsp. fresh lemon juice

- ½ cup water

Instructions

1. Chop the celery into 1 inch pieces and add to the blender along with the lemon juice and water.

2.   Blend for a minute, until the celery is completely broken down and you are left with a slurry.

3. Put a mason jar or glass in the middle of a large bowl (to minimize a mess).

4. Pour the celery slurry through a nut milk bag or cheesecloth, and use your hands to squeeze all the juice out.

5. You can discard the fiber/pulp left behind.

Cabbage juice

Preparation time

Ingredients

- 2 big sized cabbage

- Juice extractor

Instructions

1. Wash nd remove 1 layer of the cabbage in case of dryness.

2. Cut into desirable shapes so it can fit in d juicer to extract juice.

3. Serve fresh

Cranberry Coulis Recipe

Preparation time

30 minutes

Ingredients

- 6 ounces fresh cranberries (washed)

- 1 large orange (zested and juiced)

- 1/4 cup sugar

- 1/4 teaspoon ground cinnamon

- 1/4 teaspoon ground cloves

- 1/4 cup orange liqueur (Triple Sec, Cointreau, Grand Marnier)

Instructions

1. Gather the ingredients

2. In a small saucepan, combine the cranberries, orange juice and zest, sugar, cinnamon, and cloves.

3. Simmer over medium heat until cranberries burst, about 15 to 18 minutes.

4. Remove saucepan from heat, add the orange liqueur, and mix well.

5. Process in a blender or food processor until puréed.

6. Warm gently before serving.

7. Add to your Thanksgiving spread and enjoy!

Carrot and Kale Quinoa Patties

[Vegan]

Preparation time

35 minutes

Ingredients

• olive oil

• 1 1/2 cups cooked quinoa (equates to 1/2 cup uncooked quinoa)

- 2 tablespoons ground flaxseeds and 6 tablespoons of water, soaked for 10 minutes

- 1 cup kale, finely chopped (equates to approximately three leaves)

- 1/2 cup rolled oats, ground into flour (For a gluten-free patty, use gluten-free oats)

- 1/2 cup carrot, finely grated (equates to half of one large carrot)

- 1/4 cup pumpkin seeds

- 1/4 cup fresh basil, finely chopped

- 1/4 cup nutritional yeast

- 1/4 cup onion, finely diced

- equates to half a small onion

- 1 clove of garlic, minced

- 1 tablespoon tahini

- salt and pepper

Instructions

1. Preheat the oven to 400°F.

2. Line a baking tray with baking paper.

3. Heat the oil in a frying pan over a medium heat and cook the onions for five minutes or until soft.

4. Add the garlic and cook for a further two minutes.

5. Combine all ingredients, including the cooked onion and garlic, together in a large bowl. Stir well until the mixture comes together.

6. With wet hands, shape mixture into 1/4 cup patties. Pack tightly so they will hold together better.

7. Place onto lined baking tray.

8. Bake for 15 minutes then turn and bake for a further 10 minutes or until golden.

9. Allow to cool for 5 minutes then enjoy.

10. Leftovers can be stored in the fridge to up to 5 days.

11. Enjoy cold or to reheat, preheat a frying pan, and cook patties for about 3 minutes on each side in a little bit of oil.

Raw Purple Sauerkraut [Vegan]

Preparation time

5 days

Ingredients

- 1/4+ large head or 1/2 small head green cabbage

- 1/4+ large head or 1/2 small head purple cabbage

- 1-2 grape leaves

- 1-2 bay leaves

- 2-3 black peppercorns

- 1 sprig fresh or dried dill

- 4 1/2 teaspoon + pink Himalayan salt

- 1 tablespoon unpasteurized miso paste

- 1-inch fresh ginger root, peeled and finely chopped

- 4 cups filtered water

Instructions

Prepare the ingredients.

1. Sterilize your jars and lids: pour about 1 inch of water in a wide large pot and bring to simmer.

2. Place large splatter screen with a flat and even top on top of the pot.

3. Put your jars and lids upside down on the splatter screen over the simmering water. The steam should be entering the jars and you will notice water condensation inside of the jars.

4. Allow to steam for about 10-15 minutes.

5. Remove the jars and lids from pot and set on top of a clean kitchen towel upside down, so they can drain and dry.

Prepare the cabbage:

1. remove about 4-5 outer leaves from the cabbage and set aside.

2. Cut the cabbage head into quarters.

3. Using a mandoline slicer or a sharp knife, shred the cabbage into about 1/4 inch strips. Do

not shred the cabbage too thin! This may result in the sauerkraut being too soft and mushy.

4. Place the shredded cabbage in a large bowl, toss it so the purple and green cabbage are evenly mixed. Do not squish the cabbage or put any pressure on it, or it may result in a soft kraut. Set aside.

5. Fill the jars: once the jars are cool and somewhat dry (they don't have to be completely dry inside), place them on a kitchen counter with the opening facing up.

6. Sprinkle a pinch of salt on the bottom of each jar.

7. Add grape leaves, dill, bay leaves and peppercorns.

8. Place some of the cabbage mixture to a jar.

9. Using   potato masher or a large wooden spoon, gently press the cabbage down, so that it is compact but not squashed. The cabbage should not release any juices.

10. Repeat with the remaining cabbage until the jars are full, leaving about 1-1/2-inch of space from the top.

Prepare the brine:

1. in a blender, combine water, salt, miso and ginger and blend until smooth. The brine may foam and expand slightly, which is normal.

2. Fill the jars with cabbage with the brine. Give it a few minutes to release all the air (you will see air bubble rising to the top). Using potato masher or a large wooden spoon, gently press

the cabbage down. It should slightly wilt and shrink in size. You may have to add some more cabbage on top, gently pressing it down. If the cabbage is not completely covered with liquid, add some more brine. Roll the outer cabbage leaves into very tight rolls and place them on top of the mixture to fill that 1-inch space. That will serve as a spacer, so the cabbage mixture is completely submerged and has no contact with air (that is important). When you press the rolls into the jars, some of the brine will spill over, which is OK. Tightly close the jars with the sterilized lids. Place the jars on a baking sheet or a tray with raised edges on your kitchen counter or in the pantry and let ferment for 5 days.

3. Fermentation process: be sure that the room temperature is between 65° and 75°F. If it is

slightly colder, wrap a towel around each jar and keep in the pantry. If it is hotter, find a cooler place to keep your jars. During the fermentation process you will notice bubbles rising from the bottom of the jars to the top and the cabbage mixture expanding slightly. You may also hear noises and see the brine spilling out (that is why you need to keep the jars on the tray). These are the signs of the healthy fermentation process and they are perfectly normal. You may also notice smell coming from the spilled-out liquid. You can get rid of the smell by carefully placing the jars on the counter, discarding the liquid and washing the tray, then placing the jars back on it. When moving the jars, it is important to be very careful. Do not shake the jars and avoid any kind of disturbance, because that can interfere with the fermentation process. You may also notice that the cabbage mixture will shrink in size towards the end of the fermentation. This is normal as well. You should expect total shrinkage of about 10-20 percent.

4. Chilling: at the end of the 5th day, carefully wipe the outside of the jars with a damp cloth and transfer them to the refrigerator. Let chill overnight. Chilling slows down the fermentation process, but it will still be going. Once chilled, open the jar, remove the rolled outer leaves and discard. You may notice that the top layer is slightly dryer and has a different texture, which is normal. You can mix it in with the lower layers to achieve more uniformed consistency. Once the seal is broken on each jar, the sauerkraut will keep in the refrigerator for 1 month.

Cinnamon Spiced Apple and Grape Salad [Vegan]

Preparation time

20 minutes

Ingredients

• 2.5 oz herb salad mix (mix of baby lettuces, red & green chard, mizuna, arugula, friseé, radicchio, parsley, cilantro, dill, baby spinach)

• 1 tablespoon coconut oil, melted

• ½ tablespoon maple syrup

• ½ tablespoon lemon juice

- coconut oil, for cooking

- ½ cup apples, thinly sliced

- ½ cup grapes, chopped

- handful walnuts, chopped

Instructions

1. Tear salad leaves into bite-sized pieces.

2. Combine coconut oil, maple syrup, and lemon juice in small bowl.

3. Pour over salad and massage gently onto the leaves.

4. Heat a skillet on medium heat and place aprox. ½ tablespoon coconut oil in it.

5. Place slices of apple in pan.

6. Sprinkle with cinnamon.

7. Drizzle with maple syrup (optional).

8. When they begin to become golden brown and become soft, flip and pan-fry the other sides until golden brown.

9. Turn off heat and add apples to your salad bowl.

10. Place the chopped grapes into the pan, just to let them become a luke-warm temperature.

11. Combine grapes in salad.

12. Top with chopped walnuts.

13. Enjoy!

Instant Pot Cabbage Soup

Preparation time

30 minutes

Ingredients

- 2 tablespoons olive oil

- 1 cup carrots

- 1 cup celery

- 1/2 cup yellow onion

- 1 teaspoon sea salt

- 1/2 teaspoon black pepper

- 1 teaspoon Italian herb seasoning

- 3 cloves garlic, minced

- 4 cups cabbage, shredded

- 1 cup sweet corn

- 1 cup zucchini

- 4 cups vegetable broth

Instructions

1. Add oil to the instant pot and turn it on the sauté function.

2. Add carrots, celery, and onion and sauté 5 minutes until softened.

3. Add garlic and sauté 3 more minutes.

4. Add cabbage, corn, zucchini, and broth, then stir to combine.

5. Set the instant pot to soup function for 20 minutes.

6. After 20 minutes, turn the valve to instant release.

7. After pressure has released, open and stir.

8. Serve and enjoy!

Matcha Berry Pancakes

Preparation time

10 minutes

Ingredients

For the Wet Mix

- 1 tablespoon flax seeds, ground

- 2 1/2 tablespoons warm water

- 2/3 cup almond milk, unsweetened

- 1 teaspoon vanilla extract

- 1 teaspoon apple cider vinegar

- 1 tablespoon olive oil

- For the Dry Mix

- 1 cup gluten free all-purpose flour

- 1 teaspoon baking powder

- 1/4 teaspoon baking soda

- 1/4 teaspoon salt

- 1 teaspoon matcha powder

For the Pancake Garnish

• Berries

• Maple syrup

• Vegan butter

Instructions

1. For the wet mix, in a bowl mix the ground flax and the warm water and allow to sit for 10 minutes.

2. Add the almond milk, vanilla extract, apple cider vinegar and olive oil and stir well.

3. Set aside until ready to add to the dry mix.

4. For the dry mix, add the flour, baking powder, baking soda, salt and matcha to a bowl and whisk till well mixed.

5. Add the wet mix and stir until most of the lumps are gone.

6. Be careful not to over stir!

7. To cook the pancakes, heat a skillet over medium heat and add a small amount of oil to the pan.

8. Ladle out a portion of the pancake batter into the pan.

9. Sprinkle some of the fresh fruit around the top of the pancake.

10. Cook until the pancake is bubbling around the edges and then flip (after about 4 minutes).

11. Cook on the other side about 4-5 minutes or until cooked all the way through.

12. To serve, top with more berries, maple syrup and vegan butter!

Hazelnut Mousse With Warm Raspberries

Preparation time

1 hour 10 minutes

Ingredients

For the Mousse:

- 14 ounces silken tofu

- 1 handful cashews

- 1/2 cup hazelnut butter/cream

- 1/3 cup maple syrup, plus more to taste

- 1/4 cup cacao

- 1/2 teaspoon cinnamon

- A tiny pinch of salt

- 1/2 cup coconut oil, melted

For the Raspberries:

- 1/2 cup frozen raspberries

- 1 tablespoon liquid sweetener

Instructions

To Make the Mousse:

1. Mix all ingredients for the chocolate mousse in a blender until completely smooth, then taste and adjust the flavoring.

2. Run the blender again to make sure all added flavors are properly blended in.

3. Scrape into a bowl, place in the refrigerator and let cool properly for a few hours.

4. If you are short of time, please in the freezer for 45 minutes, being sure to stir it a few times during so it doesn't freeze through.

To Make the Raspberries:

1. Five minutes before serving, warm the raspberries in a pot on low heat and add the sweetener.

2. Add a couple of tablespoons of water, if needed, for easier defrosting in the pot.

3. Serve the chocolate mousse cold, topped with the warm raspberries.

Baked Kale Chips

Preparation time

20 minutes

Ingredients

- 1 Bunch Kale

- Nutritional Yeast

- Spices

Instructions

1. Preheat oven or toaster oven to 225F.

2. Tear kale into uniform-sized pieces, but don't make the pieces too small – they will shrink down.

3. Place kale on a non-stick cookie sheet or a cookie sheet lined with parchment paper.

4. Sprinkle generously with spices such as nutritional yeast, Old Bay seasoning, sea salt, garlic salt or anything you like.

5. Bake for 7-10 minutes until the kale pieces are dark green and crispy, taking care not to burn them.

Homemade Kimchi

Preparation time

24 - 48 hours

Ingredients

• 2 pounds napa cabbage, cut into 2 1/2-inch pieces

• 1 pound daikon radish, peeled, sliced thinly and cut into 1-inch pieces

- 2 seedless cucumbers, cut into 3-inch segments, then sliced lengthwise into 6 to 8 pieces

- 1 cup sea salt (non-iodized)

- 2/3 cup rice vinegar

- 1/2 cup finely chopped garlic

- 1/4 cup peeled and grated ginger root

- 1 cup gochugaru powder (see note below)

- 1/4 cup sesame seeds

- 2 teaspoons sugar

- 2 carrots, peeled and julienned into thin matchsticks

Instructions

1. Place the prepared cabbage, daikon, and cucumber in a large bowl (the biggest one you have), and toss well.

2. Sprinkle some of the salt over the top, then, wearing food-safe gloves, toss the vegetables with your hands, coating them evenly.

3. Add more salt, and toss again.

4. Continue adding a bit at a time while tossing until all the salt has been added and the vegetables are evenly coated.

5. Cover the bowl loosely with a clean kitchen towel, and let sit at room temperature for 1 hour.

6. While the vegetables are sitting, make the pepper paste.

7.   Combine the rice vinegar, minced garlic, grated ginger, gochugaru powder, sesame seeds, and sugar in the bowl of a food processor, and process until blended.

8. Scrape down the sides and process again until a thick paste forms.

9. When the vegetables are done sitting, you will notice a lot of liquid has collected in the bowl.

10. Transfer the vegetables to a strainer, and rinse them well under cold water, using your hands to toss them, ensuring that all surfaces have been evenly rinsed.

11. Let them drain briefly, then in batches, pat the vegetables dry with a clean lint-free towel.

12. Rinse and dry the mixing bowl, then place the vegetables back in the bowl, and also add the julienned carrots and the red pepper paste.

13. Wearing food-safe gloves, use your hands to toss the mixture until it is evenly mixed and every surface of the vegetables is coated with the paste.

14. Transfer the mixture to one large 8-cup jar, or a few smaller jars, packing it in tightly so no air bubbles remain, and leaving about 1 inch of space at the top of each jar.

15. Let the jars sit tightly closed on the counter at room temperature for 24 hours (or 2 days if your kitchen is chilly), then transfer to the refrigerator for storage.

16. Enjoy!

Waldorf salad

Preparation time

10 minutes

Ingredients:

- 4 large apples (use a combination of red delicious and granny smith), cored and cubed

- 4 stalks celery, chopped

- 1 cup chopped walnuts

- ½ cup raisins

- 2 tablespoons walnut oil

- 1 tablespoon apple cider vinegar

- salt and pepper to taste

Instructions:

1. Toss together the apples, celery, walnuts, and raisins.

2. In a small bowl, whisk the walnut oil with the apple cider vinegar and seasonings.

3. Pour over the salad, combine, and serve over a bed of greens.

Sautéed Mackerel

Preparation time

10 minutes

Ingredients:

- two, 1/2 pound mackerel fillets

- salt and pepper

- 2 tablespoons olive oil

- lemon juice

Instructions

1. Heat a sauté pan over high heat and add the olive oil.

2. Season the fillets and place them into the pan.

3. Cook for three to five minutes.

4. Flip and cook the other side until golden brown on the outside and flaky-white in the center.

5. Top with a squeeze of lemon.

Celery Juice

Preparation time

15 minutes

Ingredients

- 1 bunch organic Celery

- 1 cup of purified water

Instructions

1. Use 1 bunch of organic celery and cut off the
base to separate the stalks

2. Wash them in clean water to remove any debris

3. Chop the celery stalks into 1 inch pieces and place them in the blender.

4. Add 1/4 cup of purified water and put the lid on the blender.

5. Blend until smooth.

6. Place a clean nut milk bag over the mouth of a pitcher or bowl and pour the blended celery through the nut milk bag.

7. Use your hands to squeeze the celery juice through the bag.

8. Drink immediately, or feel free to make enough for 2 days (two bunches) and keep in sealed mason jar the fridge.

Cabbage Carrot Apple Juice

Preparation time

10 minutes

Ingredients

- 300 g white cabbage

- 2 medium carrots unpeeled

- 2 medium apples unpeeled

Instructions

1. Blend all ingredients together.

2. Enjoy!

Cabbage Cucumber Melon Juice

Preparation time

10 minutes

Ingredients

- 300 g cabbage

- ½ cucumber peeled or unpeeled

- ¼ honey dew melon peeled, deseeded

- Squeeze of lemon juice

Instructions

1. Blend all ingredients together.

2. Enjoy!

Cabbage Beetroot Orange Juice

Preparation time

10 minutes

Ingredients

- 300 g cabbage

- 1 large beetroot peeled

- 2 oranges peeled

Instructions

1. Juice the orange.

2. Blend the cabbage and beetroot together.

3. Add the orange juice.

4. Enjoy!

High-fibre muesli

Preparation time

15 minutes

Ingredients

- 300g jumbo oats

- 100g All-Bran

- 25g wheatgerm

- 100g dark raisins

- 140g ready-to-eat apricots , snipped into chunks

- 50g golden linseed

Instructions

1. Mix everything in a large bowl.

2. You can store this for up to 2 months in an airtight container.

3.   When you're ready to serve, pour lots of chilled milk over and let it soak for a few minutes.

Soft herb scrambled egg with asparagus

Preparation time

15 minutes

Ingredients

- 4 eggs

- 100g asparagus spear

- a knob of butter

- small handful of chopped tarragon or chervil

- slices of ciabatta , warmed, to serve

- parmesan , freshly-shaved

Instructions

1. Steam asparagus spears for 4-5 mins until tender.

2. Meanwhile, melt butter in a small pan and scramble the eggs.

3. Once the eggs are set softly, stir through the taragon or chervil and season to taste.

4. Pile the eggs on to the asparagus and hot, buttered slices of ciabatta.

5. Top with a few shavings of parmesan and serve.